CANCER

Contents:

Self-assessment

You must have often wondered, what is cancer? How is it caused? What can we do to prevent it? How is it diagnosed and treated? Well, this chapter is there to address these issues only. Having awareness about the cancer is the first step one can take in preventing it.

What is cancer?

Cancers are a group of diseases associated with abnormal growth of cells. Without any check, the disease may keep on progressing ultimately leading to pre-mature death. They can arise anywhere in the body and can affect people from all age groups, socio-economic strata and race. Cancer is the leading cause of morbidity and mortality in the world. According to data by International Agency for Research on Cancer, there were 141 lakh new cancer cases, 82 lakh cancer deaths and 326 lakh people living with cancer in 2012 worldwide. In our own country, about 4.7 lakh new cases of cancer are detected annually.

Cancer is responsible for death of about 3.5 lakh people annually in India itself.

Lung cancer is the most common cause of death from cancer worldwide, estimated to be responsible for nearly one in five deaths (15.9 lakhs deaths, 19.4% of the total). Amongst women, breast cancer is the commonest cause of death and is responsible for 5.2 lakh deaths annually. These figures are just a numerical representation of the vast damage caused by cancer worldwide.

One might want to assume that with recent rapid developments in medical sciences, the incidence and prevalence of cancer may be coming down. Sadly, that isn't so. According to WHO, within next two decades annual incidence of cancer may increase up to 220lakhs? With increase in adoption of modern lifestyle with unhealthy habits like lack of physical activity, decreased intake of fruit and vegetables, increasing use of tobacco, fast food, alcohol, etc.

the incidence of cancer is expected to further increase.

Cancer and its molecular basis

Cancer refers to unregulated and unrestricted proliferation* of cells. Clinically it is seen in the form of a growth. Neoplasm is an abnormal mass of tissue growing in an uncoordinated way and persisting even when the stimuli responsible for growth has been removed. A tumor is said to be benign when its characteristics are considered relatively harmless suggesting that it wouldn't spread to near-by or distant areas, can be operated easily and doesn't risk the patient's life significantly. Malignant tumors are collectively referred to as cancers, derived from the Latin word for crab, because they involve the tissues in a manner similar to a crab. Malignant tumor can invade and include:

destroy adjacent structures and spread to distant sites (metastasize) to cause death. Not all cancers cause death, if detected early and treated properly, some cancers can be cured.

Cancers result from certain changes at the molecular level in response to various external or internal stimuli (Figure 1).

Proliferation - rapid growth of cells. Mutation - genetic change in nucleotide sequence Carcinogens - cancer causing agents

Such genetic vegetables, increasing use of tobacco, fast food, change (or mutation*) may be acquired by the action of environmental agents or it may be inherited in the germ line. Environmental agents

Malignant neoplasms have features, such as

Physical carcinogens*- ultraviolet and ionizing radiation

Chemical carcinogens- components of tobacco smoke, aflatoxin, asbestos, arsenic etc.

Biological carcinogens - viruses, bacteria or parasites.

excessive growth, local invasiveness, and the ability to form distant metastases (Figure 2, Table 1).The various key changes that occur in a cancer cell are-capacity to proliferate without any growth signals, resistance to growth inhibiting signals, resistance to regular cell death mechanisms, formation of new blood supply ability to involve surrounding tissues, metastasis to distant organs (Figure 3) and failure in repair of damaged DNA.

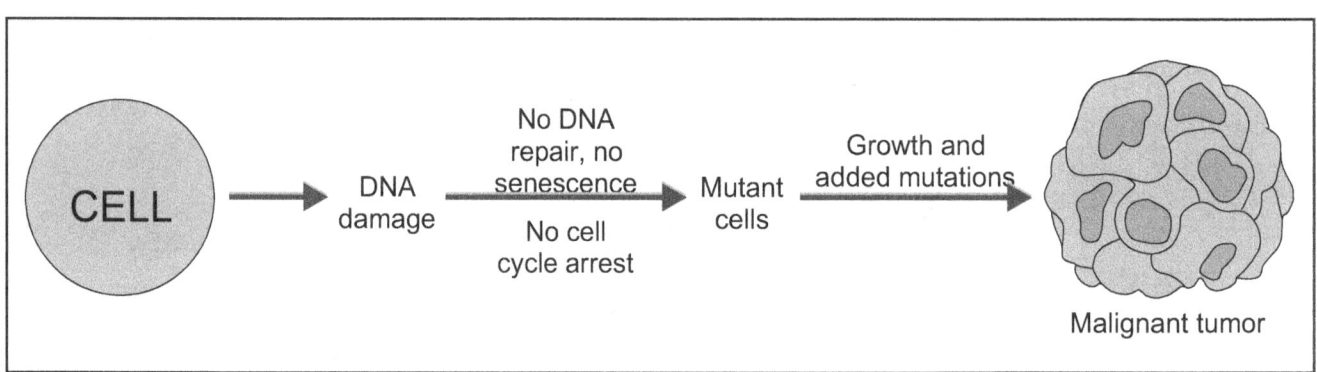

Figure 1: Simplified depiction of how a cell undergoes malignant change – with DNA damage, no repair and further mutations

Table 1: Differences between benign and malignant growth

	Malignant Growth	Benign Growth

Growth	Unregulated, fast growing	Slow growing
Surrounding Structures	Invaded or infiltrated	Compressed
Metastasis	Yes	No
Periphery	Ill-defined borders, capsule may be absent	Well-defined, Encapsulated

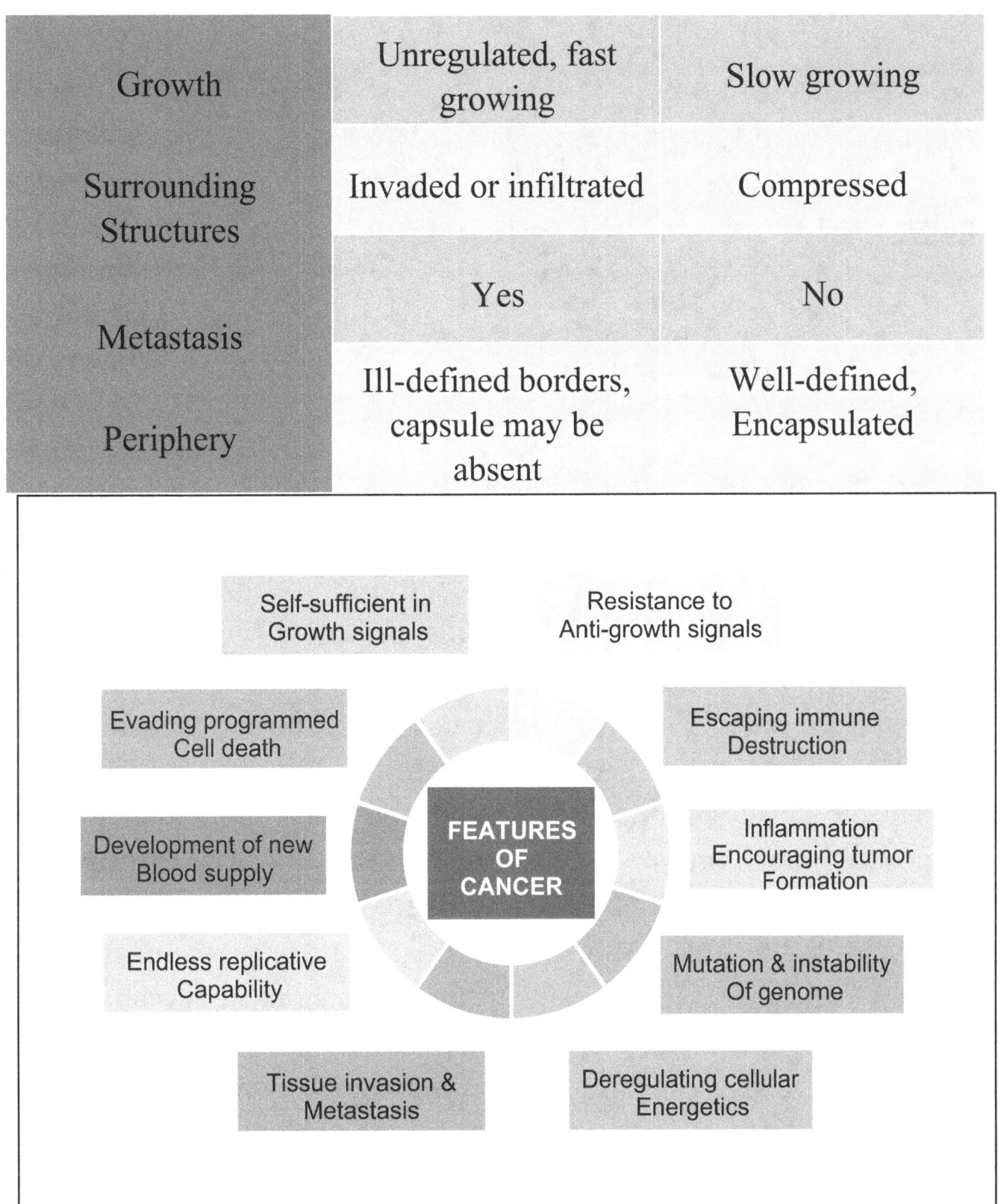

Figure 2: Features of Cancer – Major changes occurring in a cell undergoing malignant change

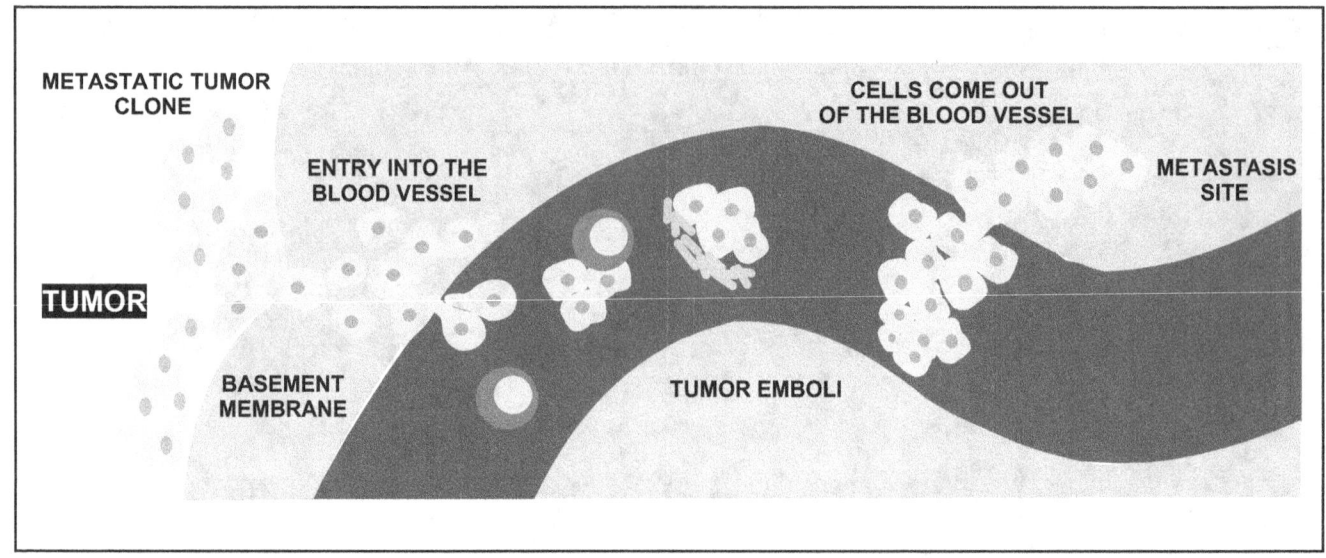

Figure 3: Schematic diagram depicting how metastasis from tumor occurs

What are the common cancers of human body? Worldwide, the commonest cancers amongst men are lung, prostate, Colo-rectum, stomach, and liver cancer. Among women the most common sites diagnosed are breast, Colo-rectum, lung, cervix, and stomach cancer. In India, amongst males common cancers in decreasing frequency are oral, lung, stomach and Colo-rectal cancers. In females, breast, cervix, Colo-rectal, ovary and oral cancers are the commonest cancers in decreasing frequency. The incidence of these cancers varies according to the geographical area, prevalent social customs and the socio-economic strata. For example, oral cancers are common in Indian sub-continent and not that common in western countries. This is because of higher consumption of chewable forms of tobacco in the form of gutkha, paan, paan masala, khaini, supari etc. Cervical cancers are commoner in women from lower socio-economic strata because of poor genital hygiene. Colo-rectal cancers occur with higher frequency in those consuming more of fatty food and less of fibbers in their diet.

What are early signs of Cancers?

Early identification of cancer is essential for proper treatment. Cancer may present in a variety of ways.

Ten common signs of cancers are:

1. New lumps or growths or swelling;
2. A sore or bruise that does not heal;
3. A mole that changes in shape, size or colour or bleeds;
4. Persistent cough or hoarseness that last;
5. Indigestion or difficulty in swallowing;
6. A change in bowel or bladder habits;
7. Shortness of breath;
8. Loss of appetite;
9. Unexplained weight loss or tiredness; and
10. Blood in urine, bowel motions or sputum.

In case of presence of any of these symptoms, the person

Figure 4: **Various causative factors associated** with cancer

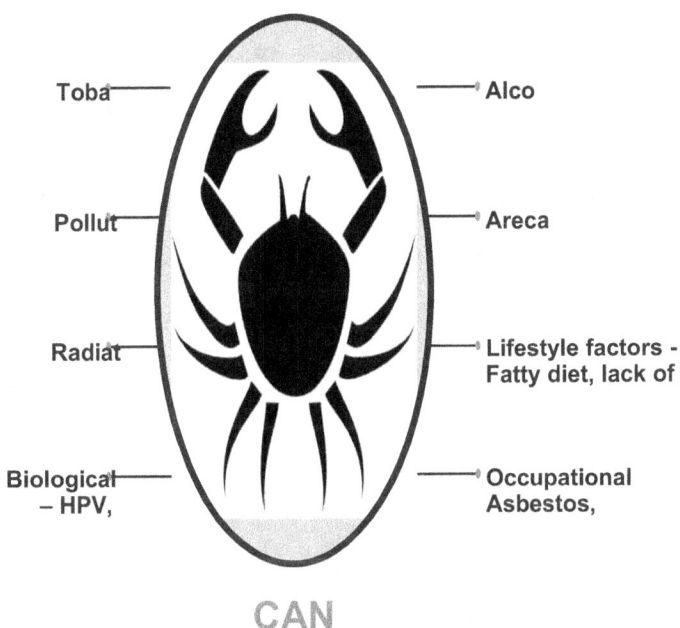

should approach the nearest doctor and get himself evaluated to rule out cancer.

What are the common causes of cancers?

Common causes of cancer are as shown in Figure 4 and are as follows:

Tobacco - Tobacco consumption is the single most important avoidable risk factor for cancer mortality worldwide. According to WHO, it causes an estimated 22% of cancer deaths per year. Majority of the lung cancers are associated with smoking. Passive smoking has also been associated with cancers in non-smoking adults. Risk increases with increasing quantity of smoking. In Indian subcontinent use of smokeless tobacco is more prevalent. These include use of Gurkha, pan masala, raw tobacco, betel quid etc. Tobacco is associated with cancers of lung, oral cavity, throat, oesophagus, urinary bladder, pancreas, kidney, liver, stomach, bowel, cervix, ovary, nose and sinus as well as some types of leukaemia (Figure 5).Tobacco contains over 4000 types of chemicals. Out of these, around 200 are harmful for human body and about 70 different chemicals have been found to be carcinogenic (Figure 6). Various studies have shown that those who quit tobacco have a better survival than those who don't. About 50% of tobacco users die because of some form of tobacco related disease. Over the counter preparations are available for nicotine replacement and these have been marketed as solution for tobacco addiction. The safety of such preparations is dubious. They have not been found to be that efficacious in curbing tobacco addiction. They themselves contain chemicals like nicotine which may cause cancer itself. A new trend, is that of the use of e-cigarettes. They are battery operated LED light containing devices which light up when used and release nicotine. They have been falsely advertised as safer alternative to cigarettes. Many studies have been conducted upon the safety of these e-cigarettes. They have been found to be associated with persistent throat irritation, seizures, pneumonia and heart failure. They contain nicotine which is highly addictive and is itself carcinogenic. Their fumes also have been found to have tobacco specific nitrosamines and other harmful chemicals. Various countries have banned or restricted the sale of such devices.

Figure 5: Common adverse effects of tobacco and alcohol

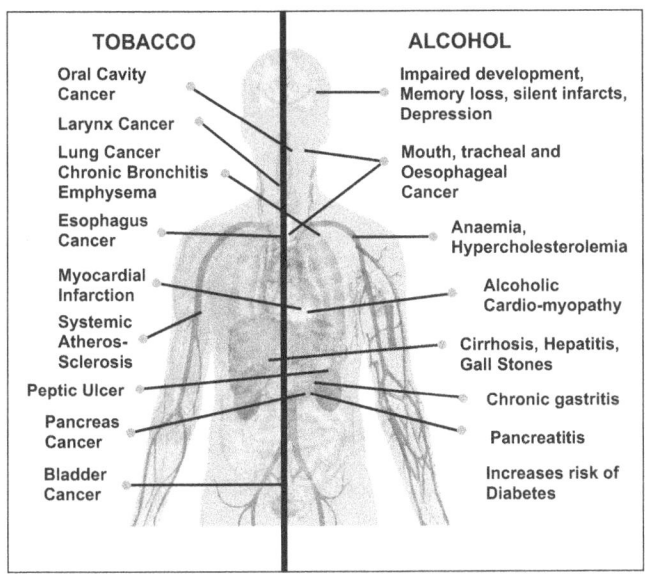

Figure 6: Harmful chemicals present in cigarette smoke

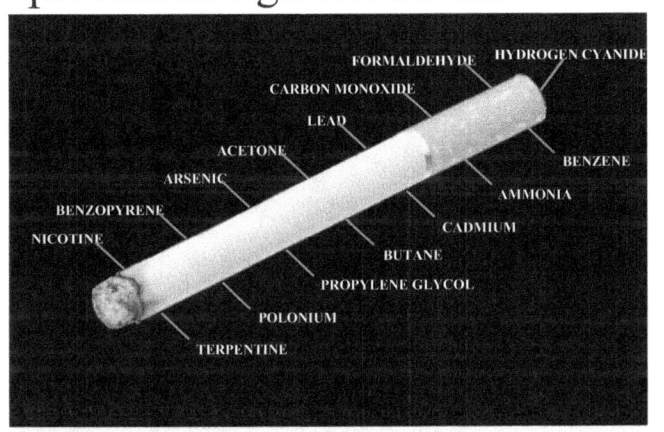

ɏ Tobacco kills around 1 million people in India each year.

ɏ Smoking causes 30% of all cancer deaths, 17% of all heart disease deaths and at least 80% of deaths due from bronchitis and emphysema.

ɏ 52.3% of adults were exposed to second-hand smoke at home.

ɏ 29.0% of adults were exposed to second-hand smoke in public places.

Alcohol: Alcohol itself is associated with several cancers, the risk of which increases with increasing quantity of alcohol consumed. It has synergistic action along with smoking and if a person consumes both alcohol and tobacco then the risk of developing cancer is much higher than the risk associated with consuming them independently. Alcohol use is a risk factor for many cancer types including cancer of the oral cavity, pharynx, larynx, oesophagus, liver, Colo-rectum and breast (Figure 5).

Areca Nut: It is also called as supari in India. It may be chewed alone or in combination with betel leaf, catechu and slaked lime – called as Pan or betel quid. Powdered areca nut in ready to eat mixtures with other ingredients is called Pan Masala. If tobacco is added to these then it is called Gurkha. It is associated with Sub Mucous Fibrosis which is a precancerous condition where the mouth opening of the chewer decreases gradually. It has been included as a group I carcinogen by The International Agency for Research into Cancer (IARC). It use has been found to lead to oral cancer. It may also result in cancers of liver and pancreas.

Pollution: This includes the environmental pollution of air, water and soil with carcinogenic chemicals. Exposure to these chemicals can occur through air and drinking water. Chemicals like arsenic cause contamination of drinking water and can result in lung cancers. Household air is polluted by coal fires and cause lung cancer. Besides, contamination of food with aflatoxins can also cause cancer.

Lifestyle factors: These include unhealthy eating habits and lack of physical activity. High body mass index is associated with cancers of esophagus, colorectum, breast, endometrium etc. Excessive consumption of red meat is associated with colorectal cancers. Healthy diet, including vegetables, salads and fruits have been found to decrease risk of developing certain cancers.

Obesity – It refers to excessive fat accumulation. If body mass index (BMI) is above 25 the person is called overweight. Those having BMI over 30 are called obese. It is associated with increased risk of heart diseases, diabetes and cancer like those of endometrium, colon, breast, oesophagus, pancreas etc. Besides increasing the risk of developing such cancers, obesity is also associated with increased chances of deaths due to such cancers. Proper healthy diet and regular exercise are required to curb the menace of obesity.

Occupational exposure: Several cancers are seen to have higher association with specific occupations. Substances like asbestos, cadmium, ethylene oxide, benzo pyrene, silica, ionizing radiation including radon, tanning devices, aluminium and coal production, iron and steel founding, have been found to be associated with various cancers. These are important to know because with adequate knowledge and precautions most of these cancers can be prevented. Common cancers associated with occupational exposure include lung, bladder, leukaemia, skin etc.

Radiation including UV rays: Ultraviolet radiation is associated with skin cancers like basal cell carcinoma, squamous cell carcinoma and melanoma*. Exposure to ionizing radiation has been associated with increased risk of several cancers. This has been extensively studied in survivors of atomic bomb in Japan.

Biological agents: These include various viruses, parasites and bacterial infections which predispose the patient to develop certain cancers. Human papilloma virus (HPV) is associated with cervical cancers and oropharyngeal cancers. Hepatitis B and C are associated with liver cancers. Parasitic (Schistosomiasis) infection is associated with increased risk of bladder cancer. *H. pylori* infection may results in stomach cancer. These infections can be prevented with precaution, vaccination and early diagnosis and treatment.

*Basal cell carcinoma, Squamous cell carcinoma and Melanoma – different types of cancer

Screening for cancer:

Screening refers to identification of a disease in an individual who has not yet developed its signs and symptoms. In this, simple tests are conducted on general population or a high risk group to identify the individuals harbouring the disease. In this way, the affected individual can be identified before he/she presents with the symptoms of the disease. Screening helps in early identification and diagnosis of several cancers. Identifying these cancers early means a better possibility of control over the disease. Screening is a useful tool in early detection of cancers of breast, cervix, oral cavity and colorectum.

Breast cancer:

Screening for breast cancer is done with mammography. Mammography refers to taking an x-ray image of the breast. Its efficacy as a screening test has been proven in several studies and it helps in reducing the morbidity and mortality associated with breast cancer. It should be done regularly in individuals having family history of breast cancer. Self-examination of breast can also help the woman to become aware about swelling in breast.

Cervical cancer:

Pap smear is used to screen women for cervical cancer (Figure 7). In this a smear taken from the cervix is evaluated under microscope to look for pre-cancerous or cancer cells. It is a cost effective method of screening. It is advisable for all women above the age of 35-40 years to undergo Pap smear examination. Besides this, visual inspection of the cervix with acetic acid application is also done at several places.

Figure 7: Schematic diagram depicting cancer of cervix

Oral cancers:

Screening for oral cavity cancers is relevant because of easy accessibility of oral mucosa for visual inspection without requiring any special equipment or expertise and the fact that most of the oral carcinomas are preceded by visible pre-cancerous lesions. Commonly seen pre-cancerous lesions include leukoplakia and erythroplakia (Figure 8). Leukoplakia refers to a whitish patch in oral cavity, for the presence of which no other cause can be found. A similar reddish patch is called erythroplakia. Biopsy from these suspicious areas may be taken to rule out malignancy.

Figure 8: Clinical photograph of the oral cavity of a tobacco chewer, smoker showing pre-cancerous and cancerous lesion.

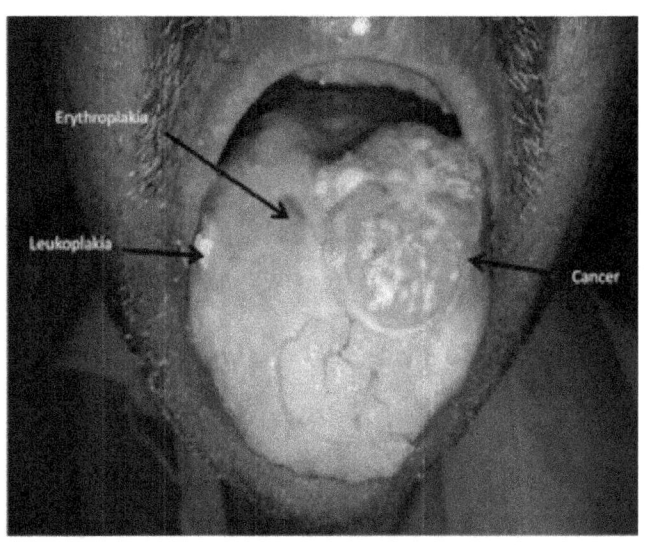

Colo-rectal cancers

Screening for these cancers is directed at people with family history of similar cancers or in those suffering from conditions like inflammatory bowel disease where there are higher chances of developing malignancy. Presence of occult blood (not visible grossly) is tested for in faeces and in certain cases colonoscopy is also done.

How is cancer treated?

Clinical examination -A patient with cancer has to be evaluated with a thorough history of symptoms and clinical examination. Endeavour is made to assess the extent of the disease and its relationship with surrounding vital structures. If required, endoscopy may be required to assess the lesion. Presence of any other disease which may affect the treatment of cancer is also looked for. Presence of any distant metastases is also evaluated.

Radiologic assessment - Clinical examination is supplemented with radiologic imaging. This may include X-ray, Ultrasonography, CT scan, MRI scan or PET scan as clinically applicable. They help in better evaluation of the lesion, its extent and presence of loco-regional or distant metastasis.

Pathologic assessment–Along-with clinical Evaluation, a small part of the lesion is biopsied* and sent for histopathological* examination. If required aspiration from the lesion is sent for cytological* examination. In both these tests, microscope and some special stains are used to assess the presence of and type of cancer cells.

Once proper clinico-radiological assessment has been done, the cancer is staged as per the existing staging guidelines. Further treatment will depend upon the type of cancer and its stage. Various modalities available are surgery, radiotherapy and chemotherapy. These may be used individually or in combination with each other as per disease status.

Surgery–Surgical excision* with reference to cancer refers to excision of the lesion with wide margins. Along with the primary lesion, regional lymph nodes are also addressed. The defect created May be closed primarily or may have to be reconstructed with local, regional or free flaps (Figure 9).

Figure 9: Operation theatre – surgery in progress

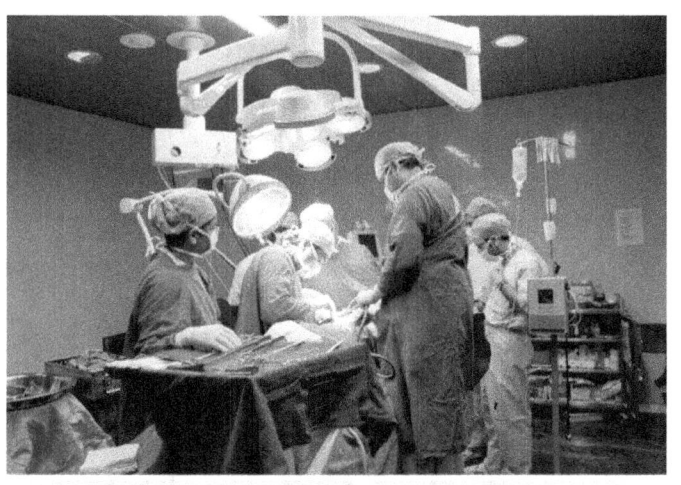

Biopsy: small part of disease is cut and sent for further examination

Histopathological, cytological examination – methods of analysing the cells under a microscope using different stains

Excision – complete removal of the disease

Radiotherapy – It involves the use of ionizing radiation for treatment of cancer. It may be used as a primary modality or as an additional therapy following or preceding surgery. Ionizing radiation acts by formation of free radicals which cause DNA damage and cell death. Radiation beam is shaped in such a way so as to cause minimum damage to surrounding normal tissues. When the source of radiation is present outside the body, it is called external beam radiotherapy (Figure 10). In some cases the source may be placed at the tumour site, in such cases it is called brachytherapy

Figure 10: A patient of cancer being treated by external beam radiotherapy using linear accelerator device

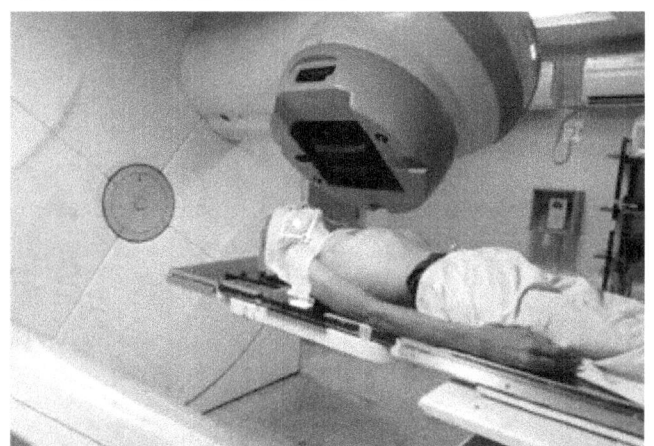

Figure 11: Chemotherapy involves administration of drugs to kill the cancer cells.

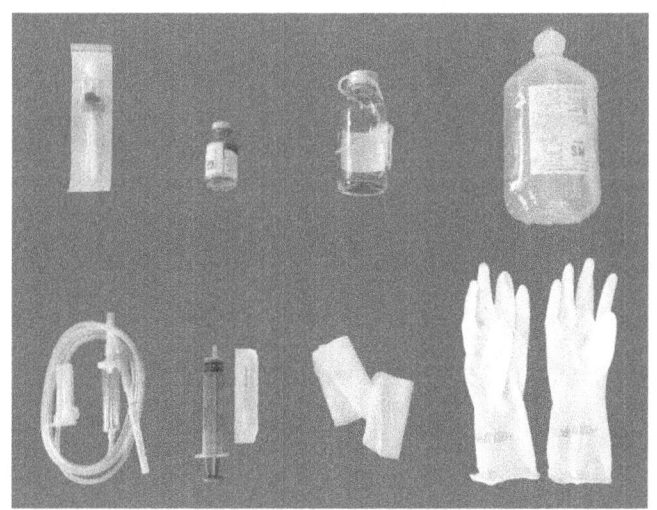

Chemotherapy – A mentioned in figure 11 a wide range of drugs are used to treat cancer. These drugs have a variety of action and act on different stages of cell cycle to cause cell death. The detail of their mechanism of action and activity is beyond the scope of this chapter. These may be used in different settings for cancer treatment. It may be the primary modality used along with radiation or may be used in adjuvant setting or also as a palliative therapy.

Palliative care – Many a time, cancer may progress beyond a stage where a curative treatment is possible. Patient may have a very advanced stage of or may have developed distant metastasis. In cases, where cure is not expected the patient is treated with a palliative intent. Palliative care involves relieving the symptoms of cancer rather than curing it. Chemotherapy or radiotherapy may be used in selective group of patients. If the general condition of the patient is very poor then he is maintained on best supportive care. Medications are given to ease of the pain and the patient is helped to carry out activities of daily living. Hospice care (institutions providing end-of-life care) may also be required in some cases.

Prevention of cancer

Towards the end of this chapter, we come onto a very important topic – prevention of cancer. What can you do to prevent cancer?

First and foremost comes – cessation of tobacco consumption. Tobacco is the single most important cause of deaths related to cancer in up to 20% of people. One should stay away from both chewable as well as non-chewable forms of tobacco. Alcohol cessation – alcohol itself is carcinogenic and also has increased carcinogenic effect when consumed along with tobacco.

Healthy lifestyle – regular physical activity along with diet rich in fruits and vegetables help in reducing the chances of developing cancer.

Good genital hygiene – maintenance of good genital hygiene along with safe sexual practices reduce the risk of infection with Human Papilloma Virus (HPV) and decrease the risk of developing cervical and oropharyngeal cancer. Vaccination against HPV infection is also available for adolescent girls. Curbing pollution - reduction of both household and outdoor pollution helps in reduction of risk of cancer. Household pollution with fossil fuels like coal can result in lung cancer. Outdoor pollution includes contamination of both air and water with various carcinogens.

Work place precautions – those involved in occupations associated with exposure to carcinogenic compounds or radiation should be provided adequate protection and should be examined at regular intervals.

Hepatitis B Virus infection can result in liver cancer. Proper precautions should be taken to prevent the spread of infection through infected blood products. Vaccination against Hepatitis B virus is also available and its full dose should be taken.

Family history – those with a family history of breast, thyroid, and Colo-rectal cancer should be aware of risk associated with their developing cancer. They should have themselves examined by a doctor and should be aware of the early signs of cancer.

Here is a list of some of the most popular herbs used in natural cancer treatments:

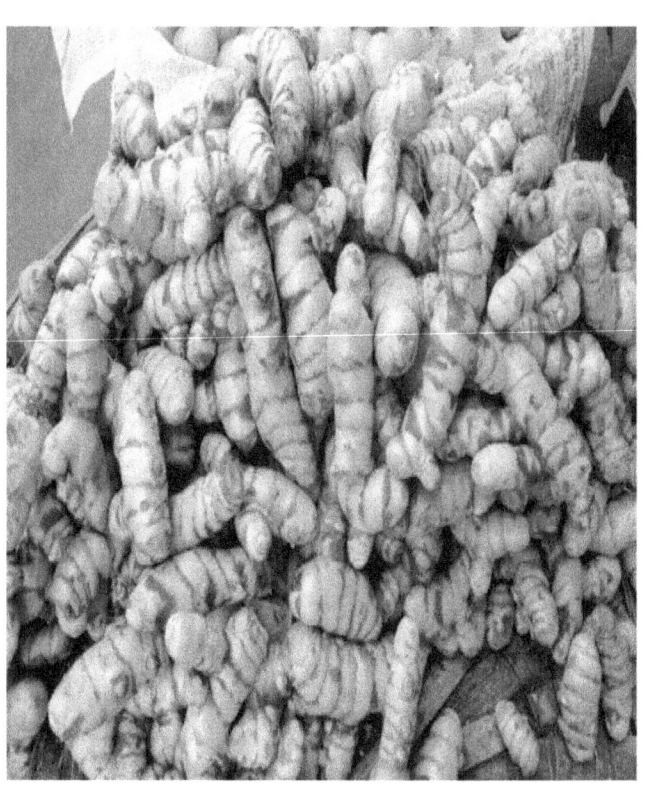

Turmeric

One of the most studied herb for cancer is turmeric, which contains the active ingredient curcumin. Curcumin possesses anti-inflammatory and antioxidant properties that can help reduce inflammation and inhibit the growth of tumors.

Cayenne pepper

Cayenne pepper contains several compounds that have been studied for their potential role in treating cancer. These compounds include capsaicin, which may have anticancer effects by inducing apoptosis (cell death) in cancer cells.

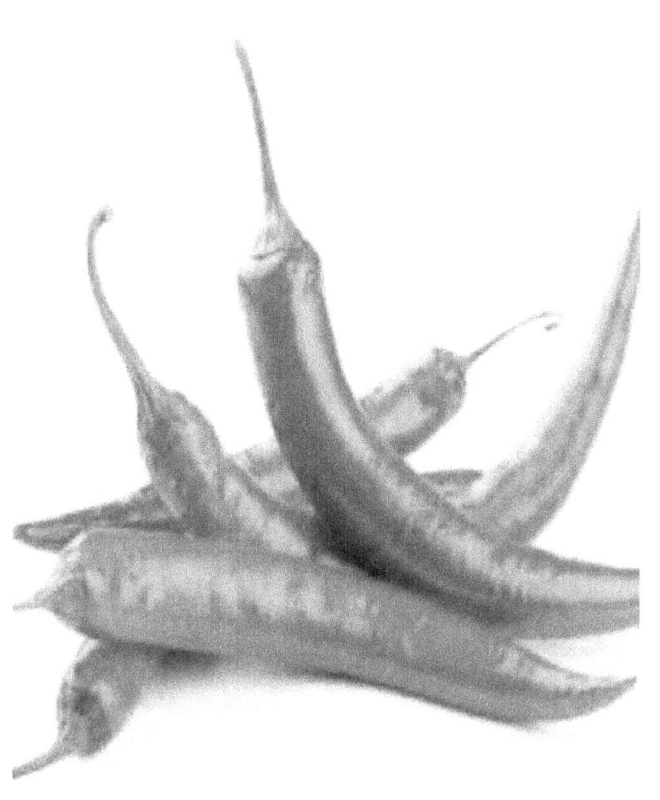

Cayenne Pepper (Shombo) - Portion
- HTSPlus

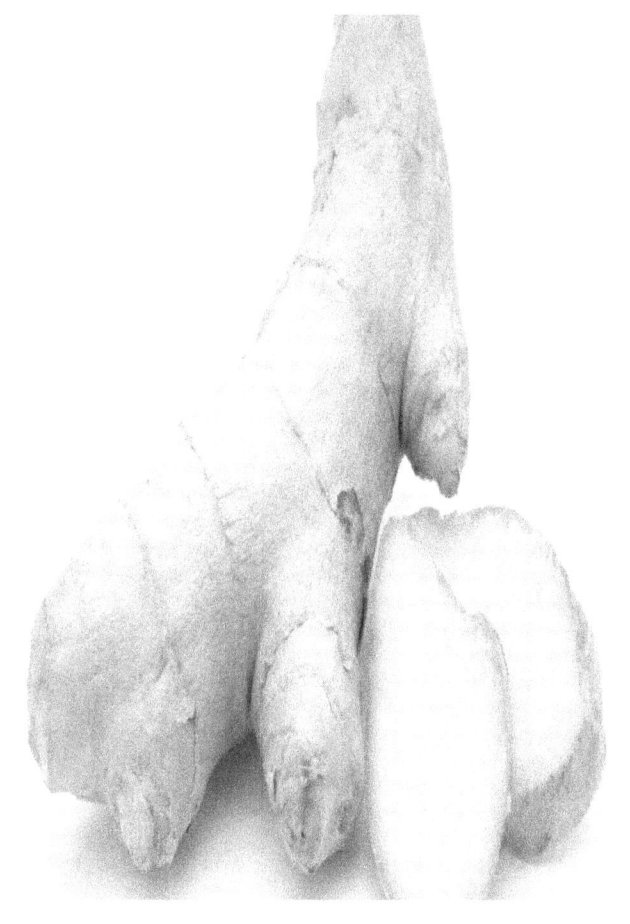

Garlic

Garlic has long been a natural remedy for many health conditions, including cancer. Studies have shown that garlic can reduce tumor growth and may help protect heathy cells from the

damage caused by **chemotherapy** drugs.

Ginger

Another popular herb for treating cancer is ginger, which may effectively reduce nausea, vomiting, and pain associated with cancer treatments.

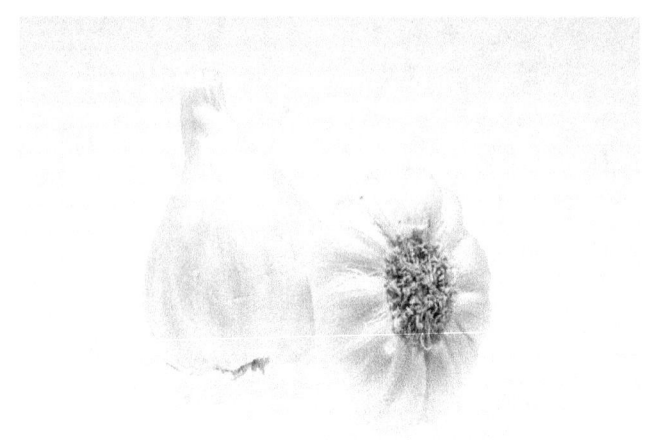

Gingko

Gingko contains compounds called ginkgo ides, which have been found to possess anti-inflammatory, antioxidant, and anticancer properties.

Echinacea

Echinacea has been used as an herbal remedy to fight infection for centuries. Recent studies have shown that it may also boost the immune system.

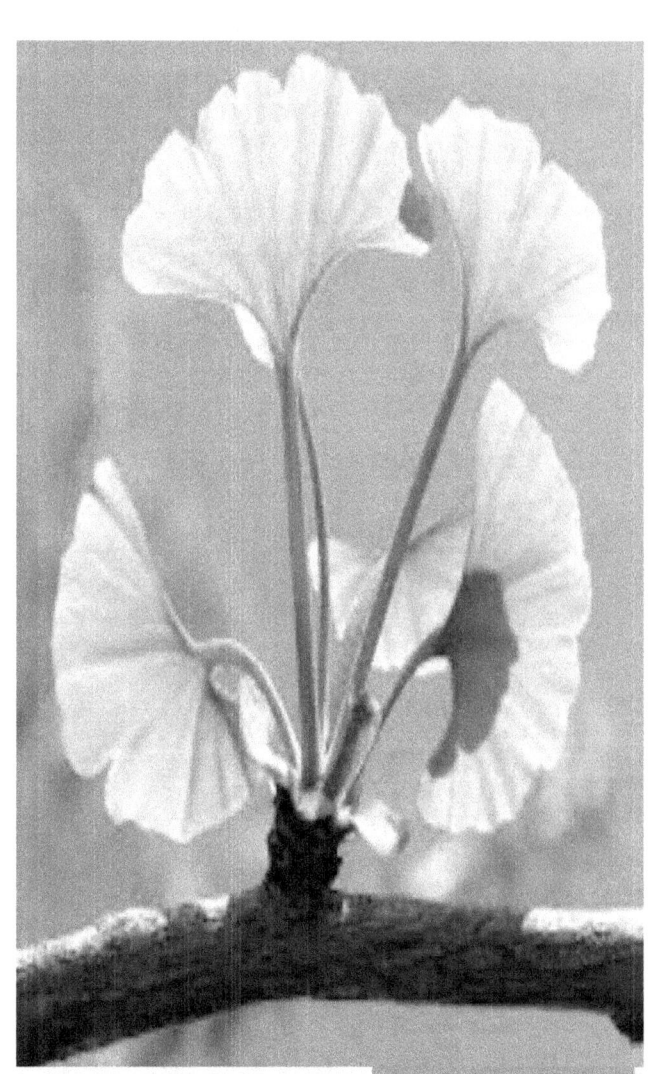

Ginkgo | NCCIH

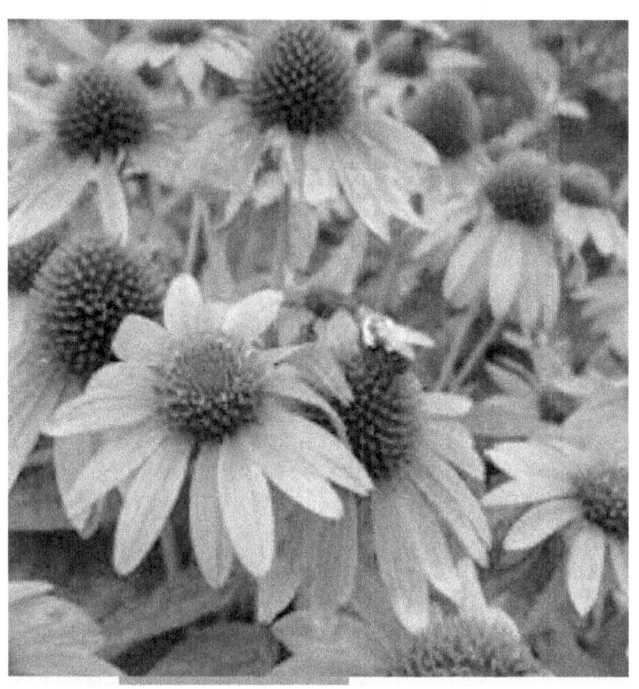

Coneflower Echinacea | HGTV

Ginseng

Ginseng is an herb that has long been used as a natural remedy to boost energy. Studies suggest it may reduce inflammation and tumor growth and protect healthy cells from damage

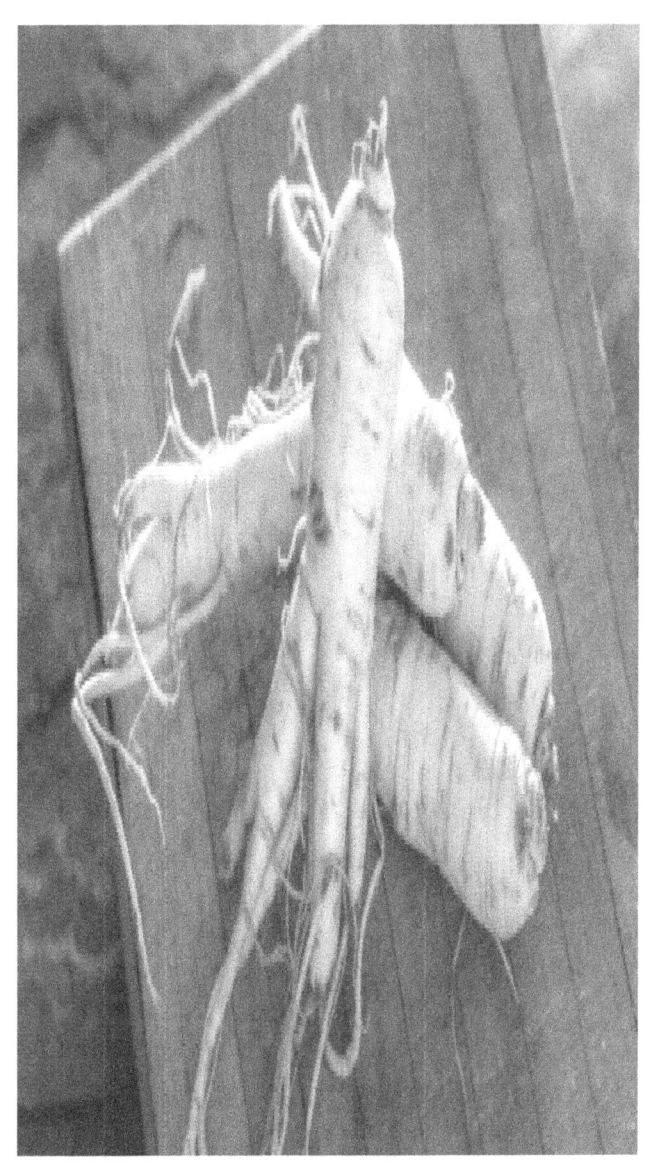

Supplements for cancer

In addition to herbs, many other natural supplements may be effective in treating cancer, including:

Omega - 3 fatty acids

Omega-3 fatty acids play a vital role in reducing inflammation and may help support cardiovascular health.

Vitamin D

Vitamin D is linked to several health benefit, including reducing inflammation.

Probiotics

Probiotics may improve digestion and support the immune system.

Vitamin E

Vitamin E is an Antioxidants that helps protect cells from damage inflammation also.

Selenium

Selenium is a mineral linked to several health benefits, including reducing the free radicals within the body that can damage cells.

Zinc

An essential mineral that helps to support the immune system, zinc may also have anticancer properties

Self-assessment
MCQ

1. **Vaccination against which virus reduces the risk of developing cervical cancer?** a) Polio

   b) HIV

   c) HPV

   d) Influenza

   Answer – c

2. **Suspicious pre-malignant white patch in oral cavity is called** a) Leukoplakia

   b) Erythroplakia

   c) Tonsillitis

   d) Fibrosis

   Answer - a

3. **Vaccination against which Hepatitis B virus reduces the risk of developing which cancer?** a) Oral cancer

   b) Stomach cancer

   c) Bone cancer

d) Liver cancer   Answer –
d

4. **Pap smear is used in screening for which cancer?**

   a) Breast cancer
   b) Lung cancer
   c) Cervical cancer
   d) Liver cancer   Answer-c

5. **Mammography is used for detection of which cancer?**

   a) Breast cancer
   b) Lung cancer
   c) Cervical cancer
   d) Liver cancer   Answer-a

6. **Most common site for cancer in males in the world is?**

   a) Breast cancer
   b) Lung cancer
   c) Cervical cancer
   d) Liver cancer   Answer – b

7. **Most common site for cancer in males in India is?**

   a) Oral cancer
   b) Lung cancer
   c) Cervical cancer
   d) Liver cancer   Answer - a

8. **Inhalation of coal smoke during household work can result in which cancer?**

   a) Lung cancer
   b) Oral cancer
   c) Liver cancer
   d) Bone cancer   Answer – a

9. **Exposure to UV rays can result in which cancer?**

   a) Brain cancer
   b) Oral cavity cancer
   c) Skin cancer
   d) Uterine cancer
   Answer – c

10. **The term 'cancer' is derived from which language?**

a) Sanskrit

b) French

c) German

d) Latin

Answer - d

2. Intake of fruits and vegetables reduces the risk of developing cancer. Answer – True

3. Supari does not cause cancer. Answer – False

4. Palliative therapy cures cancer. Answer – False

5. Use of artificial tanning machines can result in skin cancer. Answer – True

True or False

1. Exposure to radiation during childhood is associated with thyroid cancer. Answer – True